A BETTER ME

Mr. Enrique M. Tordillo Jr.
A Better Me

All rights reserved
Copyright © 2024 by Mr. Enrique M. Tordillo Jr.

Published by BooxAI
ISBN: 978-965-578-819-8

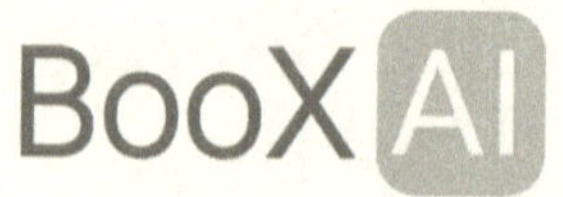

A BETTER ME

CONDITIONING YOURSELF TO LOSE WEIGHT AND STAY HEALTHY

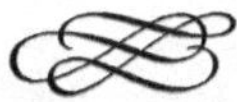

MR. ENRIQUE M. TORDILLO JR.

DEDICATION

This book is a tribute to my incredible wife, Marites Dela Cruz Tordillo, whose love has been my anchor through every high and low. To my cherished daughters, Jasmine Rain Dela Cruz Tordillo and Justine Storm Dela Cruz Tordillo, your parents hold you in the deepest of affections. In loving memory of my dear parents, Lolita Metran Tordillo and Enrique Antiquera Tordillo Sr., may their souls find eternal serenity. Gratitude fills our hearts for your presence. To all who delve into these pages, your readership is truly appreciated. Thank you for joining this meaningful journey.

CONTENTS

PREFACE

In crafting this book, my aim was to provide you, the reader, with insights garnered from both research and personal experiences. I delve into the nuances of exercising correctly, distinguishing between the right and wrong approaches. Additionally, I aim to redefine the concept of dieting and shed light on the importance of fasting in our bodies, all encapsulated in the title "Conditioning Yourself to Lose Weight and Stay Healthy: Grow Old and Healthy, my friend."

FOREWORD

Between 2017 and 2023, this book came to life as a personal journey unfolded on its pages. It all began at 45, a time when echoes of my college days reverberated vividly. Back then, I thrived in the vibrant world of the Karate Judo Team, traversing city limits for tournaments, relishing the thrill of basketball, and cherishing every opportunity to exercise. But as the years advanced, the shadows of age started casting their cloak. My body, once resilient, began to succumb to the weight of time. Weight piled up, health issues arose, and the relentless demands of family life took center stage. Responsibilities as a husband and father loomed large. Before I realized it, my health slipped through my fingers, besieged by the weight of high blood pressure, stress, and anxiety. This book encapsulates the saga of navigating these turbulent waters over six years, a narrative I share in the hope that my journey might light a path for others facing similar tides.

DISCLAIMER

I am not a certified professional. The content in this journal reflects solely my personal experiences. Prior to taking any action, I strongly advise consulting your doctor, nutritionist, or an appropriate expert. This material is intended for informational purposes exclusively.

INTRODUCTION

Get ready for a twist in this tale! To truly absorb the essence, start from the beginning, skip the middle (although you'll miss some pivotal moments), and aim for the later chapters. This book isn't about boring you; it's here to offer a vital lesson.

Let's talk priorities. Forget the luxuries like mansions and fancy cars; the real investment is in your health. After all, what's the worth of wealth if you can't savor it due to poor health? Even the well-off are recognizing this truth nowadays. When goals are achieved, it's your physical and mental well-being that truly matter.

This book won't transform you into a powerhouse overnight, but it holds the wisdom I've gained over the years to steer you towards a healthier, happier life.

It surprises me how many people still lack basic

knowledge about healthy eating and essential drinks. My hope is that this book opens minds and prompts better health choices.

Let's embark on a journey together to rewrite our story, fueled by my passion to change lives. Countless miss out on longer, healthier lives due to their habits, and it's time to rewrite that narrative.

MY JOURNEY

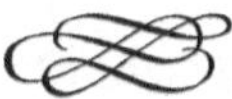

Have you ever thought about how we should get wiser as we age? It seems like common sense, right? But it's strange how we often miss the mark. The choices we make every day—what we eat and drink—should really point us towards healthier options. But instead, we tend to ignore the impact these choices have on our bodies. It's time we wake up to the fact that some of the stuff we put in our bodies is downright harmful. Let's agree that preventing obesity is within our grasp; it's a starting point to avoid a host of illnesses like diabetes, heart disease, and high blood pressure. Plus, it plays a significant role in how we feel about ourselves mentally.

My journey with exercise started when I was just ten. No strict routines, no specific plans—dieting wasn't even on my radar. But when I hit 40, things changed. Losing weight became slower, almost a puzzle. I used to joke that eating a donut and having a soda meant gaining two pounds. It baffled me for years. Even at 40, I stuck to my old beliefs—no diets, just exercise—for another six years. It turns out I was way off the mark!

At 47, I took a serious turn toward my health. I dug deep into the right way to exercise, learning the dos and don'ts. In the past, I'd often injure myself, setting my progress back. One major injury took a whopping year and a half to heal from. Lesson learned: start exercising gently, easing into it. Begin with lighter weights; let your body guide you to heavier ones. Take it slow. Start with three or five reps, and gradually increase. It's about the long-term game plan.

Have you seen those movies portraying drug addicts trying to break free from their addiction? Entering this program feels somewhat similar; bidding farewell to old habits isn't a walk in the park. It's akin to a withdrawal period—a tough phase where, as creatures of habit, we detach from the bad to embrace the good. This isn't about just exercising, dieting, or intermittent fasting; it's about self-motivation and encouragement. Change isn't a smooth ride, but believing that these changes will ultimately benefit you is a motivation in itself—an act of faith.

The phrase "You are what you eat" used to float around, and it holds true. But its interpretation can vary. Now, I resonate more with "Watch what you eat." Initially, I'd brush off hunger as just hunger. But now, through research and experience, I've discerned what's good and bad to consume—details neatly documented in my journal.

Allow me to emphasize that a healthy body breeds a healthy mind, especially when no protruding gut exists. This is a struggle for me, particularly after starting a family. Let's face it, amidst the responsibilities, caring for our bodies sometimes takes a backseat, especially for middle-class families hustling to make ends meet. However, this book serves as your compass to self-care and health. It's your roadmap back to a better version of yourself if you ever veer off track.

The perennial questions about weight loss, shedding belly fat—everyone's got them. Let me walk you through my journey of shedding weight, losing belly fat, and conquering my bad habits along the way.

We humans are fortunate to have choices, unlike our animal counterparts. But within this plethora of options lie some that can harm us, either due to our conscious decisions or our unawareness of their health implications. Through this book and my life experiences, I aim to shed light on these choices, empowering you to make healthier decisions.

I grappled with weight loss for years, trying different methods and routines, only to end up back where I started. This led me to question: What was I doing wrong? I took the time to map out my journey and researched extensively. Everything I learned, every success and every misstep, is now documented in this book to guide you through similar challenges.

Dealing with diet, exercise, and intermittent fasting isn't easy. It's common to hit plateaus that can last for months, but persistence is key. Your body might just need time to adapt to new habits. Stay patient, stay positive. Slow progress is better than undoing all your hard work. Take a moment to understand why your progress might be slow. Assess your food choices and consider mixing up your workouts.

YouTube became my go-to for weight loss knowledge. It's a treasure trove for learning about specific body parts and what works best. Watching dos and don'ts saved me from making mistakes. Doing things right from the start saves time—I've learned that the hard way.

Breaking old habits, especially when it comes to unhealthy eating and drinking, is a challenge. I struggled with alcohol and took years to overcome it, gradually reducing consumption and replacing it with tea or water during cravings.

Starting small is essential. I began my exercise journey with basic stretches in the first week to loosen up my stiff muscles. It's like preparing the body, oiling its joints, for the journey ahead.

Food not to eat or food/drinks that can make your stomach bloat:

1. Any soda
2. Any beer
3. Any junk food
4. Milk
5. Fried food
6. Ice cream
7. Anything with sugar, especially donuts.
8. Rice. (Yes, I said it, Rice)
9. Bread
10. Power drink
11. Spicy food

From personal experience, I gradually phased out certain foods and drinks rather than cutting them off abruptly. Some items are easier for me to avoid than others.

Late-night snacks can contribute to extra body fat. I try my best to steer clear of them, but when cravings strike hard, I opt for something light and follow it up with water to trick my stomach into feeling full.

Initially, I believed that rigorous cardio, abs workouts, and running were all I needed for fitness. But as I aged, I realized this wasn't the whole picture. Despite intense workouts, I struggled to lose my belly until I altered my diet—voila! Results and even six-pack abs followed suit.

Shedding unwanted weight has numerous perks: feeling and looking better, heightened stamina, and improved overall health. It enhances productivity and translates into positive mental vibes originating from a healthier core.

Though I dine out frequently, I steer clear of desserts like pastries or ice cream, opting for fruits instead—cantaloupe, grapes, watermelons—the natural sweetness satisfies the craving.

So, when the sweet tooth strikes, I grab fruits—seedless grapes, sweet apples, cantaloupes, oranges, mangoes, and watermelons. Eventually, I stopped eating before bedtime, practicing an intermittent diet.

High cholesterol is one of my medical concerns. While my doctor suggested medication, I've found that reducing egg consumption significantly helped. This is purely based on my personal observation and experience.

Let's be honest: resisting food temptations and bad habits isn't easy—this is where many falter. But for those who succeed, the reward is immeasurable, akin to the definition of insanity: expecting different outcomes from repetitive actions. That, my friend, is truly crazy.

Embarking on this journey while juggling a full-time job plus an extra four hours on some days (yeah, even on my supposed days off!) isn't a cakewalk. I rush from work, swap my uniform for workout gear, squeeze in a solid hour and a half of exercise, scarf down a quick bite, shower, and hit the hay—it's a whirlwind!

On my off days, it's game on! I dive into a full workout extravaganza lasting two to three hours. Think abs, cardio, arm workouts—the whole shebang. I wish I could promise this every week, but hey, life's about giving it your all, right?

Let me tell you about this game-changer—a $20, 8-pound vest from Walmart. It's like a magic trick! Strapping it on during runs and warmups melted away a whopping 10 pounds of body fat in just two weeks. Who knew those 8 pounds could feel like 25 over time?

The struggle is real, trust me. But when I hit those moments of wanting to throw in the towel, I remind myself of folks who've faced unimaginable challenges—people who lost limbs but never lost their fight. If they can push through, why can't I? Cue Michael Jackson's "Man in the Mirror"—my anthem when I need a lift.

YouTube is my go-to motivation hub—search for inspiring speeches or speakers. Admiral William H. McRaven's Commencement Address? Pure gold. Plus, there's Eric "ET" Thomas, Les Brown, Norman Vincent Peale ("The Power of Positive Thinking"), and Rhonda Byrne ("The Secret"). They've shaped my mindset big time!

Changing habits and the way we think? It's a rollercoaster, but these influencers have been my compass on this wild journey.

What's the endgame here? It's all about prepping for a kick-ass retirement—picture me, carefree and healthy, without relying on meds because I prioritized my health earlier in life.

And let me tell you, the perks of aging healthily? Huge! Imagine saving a truckload of meds and actually enjoying those golden years to the fullest—no health baggage weighing you down!

SUPPLEMENTS

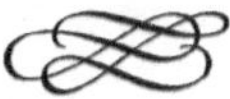

I used the Optimum Nutrition Brand for my supplements: GOLD STANDARD 100% WHEY PROTEIN ISOLATES AND BCAA. I used it before and after workouts. I mix creatine HYDROCHLORIDE POWDER with my water when I'm at work. I also take MELATONIN to help me sleep. I have a sleep problem; it's really hard for me to sleep even when I'm tired, so I take it.

I don't know any of these supplements; I just learned them from watching YouTube. I know that Whey Protein and BCAA help your muscles recover much faster, not like feeling I got run over by a truck the following day. This is just a recommendation you don't have. You can take a light exercise, and as long as you are moving or active every day, that is what counts.

I hit the gym because I was exhausted from feeling exhausted. Dealing with extra weight and nagging aches, I knew a change was overdue. Exercise seemed like the key —I was determined to nail it this time, step by step. At 46, watching my waistline expand and battling those pesky love handles, I was on a mission to bid them goodbye forever. But here's the kicker: despite all the sweat from cardio, it wasn't cutting it. I had to dive deep into the world of dieting—what to eat and, more importantly, what to avoid. This round, I was dead set on learning from past slip-ups and steering clear of them.

Here's a tidbit from my workout journey: I used to down a mix of vitamins—C, D, and Multivitamins—alongside protein powder every day. But let me tell you, the side effects were brutal. So, I made a switch. Post-workout, it was goodbye to the vitamins and hello to a protein powder-water combo. It turns out that that protein-packed potion turbocharged my muscle recovery and jolted my energy levels. For anyone struggling with similar issues, I hope this trick does wonders for you, too!

QUOTES

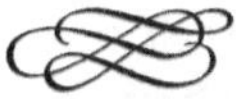

1. Fortune favors the Brave.
2. Fall 10 times, get up 11 times.
3. Thomas Edison Failed 1000X before he could invent the light bulb.
4. When One Door Closes, One Door will Open.
5. Ying and Yang. Day and Night.
6. Take that Unbeaten path.
7. Now, faith is the substance of things hoped for. The evidence of things not seen.
8. This body is just our vehicle to get to our destination; how we use this body is up to each individual.
9. Don't waste your tears on someone that doesn't love you.
10. The principles are simple but not easy.
11. Turn your Negative into Positive.

12. Make time when there is No Time.
13. Successful people don't look at their current situation; successful people look at their future situation.

I may not be an expert, but let me tell you, this recommendation that reshaped my life—helping me shed weight and transform my whole outlook—was a game-changer. If I wanted to be healthy and, let's admit it, look good (cue the laughter!), I had to change my approach. It's our mindset that propels us towards our goals; a shift in thinking can truly overhaul our lives. Ever had a phrase stuck in your head? For me, it's "take that unbeaten path." Strange, right?

Age doesn't matter when it comes to becoming a better version of yourself. This book isn't solely about health; it's about enhancing your entire being. Health, relationships, lifestyle, sports—any change can lead to a better YOU. It's within reach; you just need to rise and chase it. Nothing in life falls into our laps; it's up to us to make it happen. That, my friend, is called determination. We all desire something, and to reach it, we must truly WANT it. It's tough, but the rewards? Absolutely priceless.

I had this pile of exercise gear gathering dust for years. Does that sound familiar? Every time I passed by, I'd promise myself, "Next year, I'll make time for it." One of my excuses? "I need to catch my favorite TV show." So, what did I do? Eliminated the excuse—I set up a small TV in front of my treadmill. Running while catching up on my show became my routine; problem solved. Then came the lack of determination. Solution? While doing my exercises, I tuned in to motivational speakers on YouTube —Eric "ET" Thomas, Dr. Norman Vincent Peale, and Les Brown. These three speakers molded me into who I am today.

Visualizing our health and personal goals is key. Find exercises that suit your body and focus on the areas you want to improve. Even if it's just one pushup today, aim for two next week and three the week after. Progress takes time, but with perseverance, you'll get there. Stay positive.

I've witnessed too many people take shortcuts in losing weight only to gain it all back. Some resorted to surgeries, plunging into debt, only to regain the weight. Truly losing weight requires patience and learning to combat urges— whether it's food, drugs, or anything else. It's a step-by-step battle you can conquer.

EXERCISE

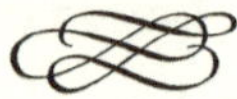

Once you start this journey, you have to commit to it; what I mean by that is you can bend it, but you have to stay with it; as I said, it takes time to change, but you will notice along the way that the sacrifice and changes are worth it and the next thing you know it that bad habits or whatever you're trying to change are gone. So let's START.

Warmups:

1. Neck roll/Head roll.
2. Head look left/right, up down.
3. Shoulder roll front/back.
4. Shoulder roll arm forward/backward.
5. Shoulder roll extended arm side forward/backward.

6. Chest: arm bent front, move forward then backward.
7. Waist roll left, then right.
8. Upper torso twist left right.
9. Side-bent right arm up, bent toward left, then switch-arms.
10. Hold something for balance, pull the left leg from the back using the right hand, then switch.
11. Hold something for balance, pull the left leg from the front using the right hand, then switch.
12. Pull left knee toward chest using both hands.
13. Pull right knee toward chest using both hands.
14. Pull the left leg back using the left hand.
15. Pull the right leg using the right hand.
16. Hamstring stretch 12X.
17. Hamstring and Thigh stretch, sit like a frog from your toes, hold on to something in front of you, and rock your left and right sides.
18. Leg stretch bent left and right side.
19. Squat.
20. Push up.

SUBSTITUTE FOR ALCOHOL

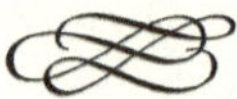

Swap out alcohol for lemon water or just plain water when you're settling in to catch your favorite TV show. Not only will you feel fuller, but you'll sidestep the urge for alcohol, saving both time and money. Plus, you can focus better on your show.

Rather than reaching for junk food, opt for healthier snacks like apples, grapes, bananas, or oranges.

About a year and a half into this journey, I faced a struggle. The temptation to indulge hit hard, so I grabbed a bottle of red wine and some pretzels to unwind after work on a Friday. As I relaxed in front of the TV and sipped my second glass of wine, I balanced it out with a couple of glasses of water. Surprisingly, even though I indulged a bit, I managed to avoid fatty foods like I used to at buffets. That weekend, I lost weight despite having some wine—it was all about steering clear of the fatty stuff.

There'll be days when you're not in the mood to work out, not because you're unwell or tired, just because. If you've skipped a couple of days, start small. Hit the gym and do half of your usual routine; you'll feel better afterward.

This isn't a quick-fix program; taking drastic steps like cutting out sugar entirely could backfire. Depriving your body might make it rebound and regain the hard-earned weight. Take your time, stay on track, and focus on better health.

At a year and seven months in, I felt myself slipping. Eating less and skipping workouts made my midsection less toned. It was time to wake up and hit the gym before I strayed from my goal. I had just eight pounds to lose, and I didn't want that number to double. Looking back, I now know which foods to steer clear of to avoid regaining that weight.

Self-discipline, motivation, and mindset can pave the way to your goal, no matter what you're aiming for.

Despite a few weeks of struggle juggling health and work issues, I managed to squeeze in workouts at least two to three days a week. Instead of shying away from my routine, I used it as a way to relax and focus amidst the chaos. I've been striving to maintain healthy eating habits through it all.

Let's talk about faith—not religiously, but in terms of visualizing what we want to achieve. If you can believe in the possibility and achievability of your goal, it becomes more tangible. Otherwise, why bother? It's all about believing in ourselves.

Can we lose weight? Absolutely. Is it attainable? Definitely. Do you need surgery or the gym to shed those pounds? No, you don't. You can do it right at home. Remember, weight loss is primarily about diet—90% diet and just 10% exercise.

Believe that you can and you will. This book advocates starting slow, allowing both your body and mind time to adjust. Embracing change isn't always easy, but once you do, the incredible results will speak for themselves. You'll look back and say, "Wow! I did it!" The journey might have been tough, but now you know what's best for your body.

Discipline and self-motivation play a pivotal role in making life changes, and with this book, you've got a compass. Whenever you veer off course from your diet or exercise, refer back to this guide. Check your progress chart from a month ago—assess where you were then and where you stand today. Ask yourself: How can I better myself? What improvements can I make? There's an answer for everything; ask around, hit the internet for research—it's all at your fingertips, and it's free.

Here are actionable steps to aid weight loss:

- Park farther away to get more steps.
- Opt for stairs over the elevator.
- Avoid heavy meals before bedtime; consider fruits if you're hungry.
- Aim for at least an hour of daily exercise, accompanied by music or audiobooks, to distract yourself. You'll find yourself done in no time.

A week has passed since my last entry; I've halted workouts due to a painful groin-like injury from my rigorous work schedule. Perhaps it's time to ease up a bit despite missing the workouts. Fortunately, I've stuck to my diet, mostly having fruits for dinner, and surprisingly, I've not gained any weight. My stomach feels great, but I miss the exercise routine dearly.

This book isn't just random advice; it's derived from years of personal weight loss experience. It's an authentic journey that led me to where I am today—a journey that works.

About a year into exercising, I shed 20 pounds, but my stubborn love handle persisted. A YouTube binge one night introduced me to a couple focused on defining their abs. That's when I learned about the right diet and exercises I needed. Within two weeks, I saw a remarkable change—it catapulted me to a different level of fitness.

In the 18th month of this journey, I've dropped 32

pounds. Although I'm close to my 40-pound goal, it feels both near and far. Injuries have slowed me down to just 2 to 3 workouts a week, mostly 2. It's time to regain focus and rekindle that determination.

Working seven days a week with overtime Sunday through Thursday is no joke. Squeezing in my workout routine amidst this hustle is a real challenge, but I refuse to let my age dictate my capabilities. My body might not bounce back as fast from weightlifting, but I'm considering upping my protein intake. Positivity is key—I still have plenty of energy left in this tank.

Recent revelation: Cold drinks make my stomach bloated! Who knew? Mixing warm food with cold drinks leads to a gassy situation, and that gas gets trapped in the belly.

Back in 2019, on November 25, I dipped my toes into a plant-based diet—not fully committed, but testing the waters, as they say.

It's been a while since I jotted something down. I'm writing now because I slipped up today. The last time I drank was back in February; I promised myself I wouldn't again, yet here I am, almost done with my 9th drink. Not a regular drinker, thankfully. I'm 47, and my stamina's impressive, but my alcohol resistance? Not so much. Put a cap on it at 9 1/2 cans, and I'm calling it a day.

Fast forward to December 2020 amidst the COVID-19 chaos; I'm now 48 and striving to keep up with workouts.

Learned a thing or two in the last few months—like bread doesn't sit well with my stomach. Tough realization for a bread lover like me, but my stomach's thanking me for it.

Lately, I've adopted the 90% Diet and 10% Workout approach. Prioritizing diet over exercise seems to be maintaining my weight as I age. Bread's on the avoid list now, though not entirely banished—just an occasional treat. Swapping out morning bread for oatmeal has been my go-to breakfast fix.

March through December amidst this pandemic has been rough. Injuries and sickness interrupted my workout routine multiple times. It's become clear: If I'm aiming to shed weight, the 90% focus on diet might just be the game-changer I need, more than the 10% on exercise.

I can't stress enough the benefits of taking Creatine and BCAA 2:1:1 after a workout. The quantity depends on how intense your session is. For a rigorous workout, I go for two capsules of creatine and BCAA 2:1:1 before and after exercising. On lighter days, it's just two capsules post-workout. Speaking of sleep, I often grapple with insomnia, so I opt for Melatonin. It's a suggestion, though, not a must if sleep isn't an issue for you.

Now, January 1, 2022, rolls in; I've been on vacation recently. My mission: bid farewell to my pesky love handles. My plan was to put in a solid 2 hours of workout daily, which I mostly did. But I realized I missed two crucial points: cutting down on SUGAR and ditching FRIED FOOD. Next weeks at work might make this tough, but I'm determined to tackle these challenges.

Fast forward to January 25; I've axed desserts and trimmed my food intake during breaks. Just one meal instead of three and lighter dinners like fruits or chicken ramen with eggs. Surprisingly, I felt great and lost 4 pounds too. My mental game is crucial in this.

Ever heard the "Know your why?" tale by Shannon Sharp? It's got some wisdom to it.

February 16, 2022 update: Dessert-free life is the real deal for me this year, day or night. Fruits have become my go-to evening snack. But alas, pollen allergies hit hard, limiting my workouts to 2 or 3 times in six weeks. On the bright side, my stomach's thanking me for skipping sweets and opting for fruits at night.

A recent show struck a chord with me when a lady mentioned, "We are what we eat," emphasizing the pivotal role of agriculture in humanity's future. It reminded me of a college quote: "An ounce of prevention is better than a pound of cure."

When I started this book, my goal was to share insights from my health journey. I've learned plenty amid weight fluctuations and the allure of tempting, unhealthy foods. Whenever I lost focus, this book became my guide, a reminder of why I chose a healthier path—a structure I crafted for myself.

Consistency is key—it's the daily effort that drives the desired outcome. Thirty minutes of exercise daily equates to noticeable results—consistency is the magic ingredient.

Fast forward to March 18, 2022: my allergies are gone, but my work schedule's been relentless, leaving little time for exercise. However, my diet's been on point, with nightly fruits boosting my morning energy. I hope to sustain this routine.

As of March 21, 2022, impatience nudges me to refocus on my abs despite my demanding work hours. It's challenging, but I'm up for the task, aiming to avoid falling ill again.

Note to self: sugar, spicy foods, and condiments can cause bloating. Listening to your body is essential—never ignore its signals.

April 22, 2022 update: To battle that persistent gut, I've invested in CLA and SST PERFORMIX from Vitamin World. I've had success with SST PERFORMIX before and plan to incorporate it again. Additionally, I've resumed my workout regimen, pairing it with BCAA, Creatine, and Protein Powder supplementation. Time to see how this combination fares this time around!

The first time I tried CLA and SST, it felt like I was buzzing with energy, but man, I couldn't sleep that night. Note to self: don't take it before bedtime. Oh, and a friendly heads-up: those bathroom trips increased dramatically, too. It could be a side effect. Let's see how this goes in the next few days, shall we?

Quick update: CLA and SST are no magic pills. They only kick in when you pair them with diet and exercise. Lesson learned—save your cash if you're not committed to sweating it out.

Guess what? I ended up testing positive for Covid-19. Crazy, right? The symptoms hit hard, especially messing with my breathing. Climbing stairs felt like climbing mountains. But hey, after a week of rest and recovery, I finally tested negative. Thank goodness for staying fit—my stamina pulled me through.

Fast forward to July 01, 2022—back on the workout grind, starting slow and steady. Changing up my diet, too—no more late-night snacking. And you know what? After just a week, I'm feeling the changes, even though my muscles are giving me a bit of a grumble with this new routine.

DIET AND EXERCISE

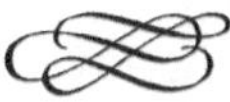

Embarking on the journey of diet and exercise, here's a truth bomb: feeling worse before feeling better is part of the process. No sugar-coating here!

July 01, 2022, update: Diet's on track, but exercise took a detour. Blame it on my kid's schedule—parenting duties come first! But here's the thing I've discovered about intermittent fasting: skipping bedtime bites isn't that bad. Think about it: Do you really need to fuel up when you're catching Zs? Your body's resting, after all. And when morning rolls in, chow down guilt-free. Your body craves it, and you burn it all day. Nighttime? Nah, your body's in rest mode.

Fast forward to September 22, 2022—exercise has taken a backseat, but intermittent fasting is still my go-to. Water and hot tea are my buddies at night, and guess what? I've been holding onto my weight. Busy days even chip off a few pounds!

October 02, 2022, I worked an insane 11-day stretch, and guess what caught up to me? Low sugar levels. So, yep, bedtime snacking made a comeback, and my gut paid the price—sugar's no joke.

Age may be just a number, but here's a lesson learned at 50: too many pre-sleep drinks mean non-stop bathroom trips. Note to self: hydration's cool, but moderation, please.

Sugar equals bloat—no ifs, ands, or buts.

November 13, 2022, back from a month's vacation and a seven-pound souvenir. Not bad for daily indulgence! Time to buckle up, aiming to get back in shape before the next holiday getaway. Intermittent fasting is back on the menu, cutting down meat intake by 70%. Tough, but hey, it's a money-saver and a weight-shedder.

But guess what? A cold and flu welcomed me home. Working those long hours didn't help, so I had to call in sick on day four. Rest, medicine, and no lifting weights— definitely not what I planned post-vacation.

You wouldn't believe it! As of 11/29/2022, I'm finally on the upswing! The cold's hanging around a bit, but the fever's waving goodbye. Step by step, I'm inching back to full health. When you're under the weather, it's all about guzzling fluids—tons of water and my go-to pulpy orange juice—plus munching on whatever helps you feel human again. The diet can wait; right now, it's about recharging those energy reserves.

Alright, picture this: I stumbled onto this epic Arnold Schwarzenegger story on TikTok. At 75, someone asked him why he was still pumping iron. His response was gold: "Why eat today when you ate yesterday? It's a habit, and it's what keeps me happy." Got me thinking—maybe the real magic is in the routine itself.

Fast forward to 12/05/2022, and I'm officially back in the game! The flu's history, and straight after a grueling 11-hour workday, I hit the gym. What is the plan now? It's not just about eating right and working out; I'm throwing intermittent fasting into the mix. And get this—current weight: 176 pounds.

Now, let's break it down: exercise, diet, and fasting. But wait, in this first month, I might give fasting a breather. Why? 'Cause I'm focused on rebuilding my strength. It's been six days since I hit the grind, and oh boy, those muscles and stamina are making a comeback. The soreness and my newfound love for water? Signs I'm crushing it. I'm not a big water fan, but now it's my secret indicator of burning fat and building muscle. Feeling the burn and fatigue? Yep, it's tough, but I'm living by the mantra: "Strike while the iron's hot" and "No Pain, No Gain." Trust me, waking up might feel like a mission, but the rewards are off the charts.

Yep, right now, I feel like I've wrestled a train—aching back, tired to the bone, arms and legs giving me attitude. But guess what? My spirit? Untouched. I'm on fire!

Remember, when you're starting anew, take it easy. Don't go too heavy on the weights right off the bat—you risk injury by overdoing it. Start light, maybe with just 10 minutes of exercise a day, then gradually add more time as you go along.

Let's rewind a bit to give you a quick rundown of my latest diet. Breakfast? A cup of coffee mixed with creatine, BCAA, and protein powder, plus a small bite—maybe a peanut butter sandwich or something quick. Oh, and while sipping on that coffee, I pop my daily vitamins: C, D, E, and a trusty multivitamin.

You know that whole "If I knew then what I know now" spiel? This book is kinda like that. I hope whoever reads this opens their mind to the idea that changing habits can make you a healthier, happier person. Just heard a co-worker's going in for a kidney transplant. Years ago, I'd see him munching on microwave meals daily and think, "Doesn't he know that's not great for him?" Maybe he didn't, and now he's paying the price. That's why I'm here—to help folks make better choices about what they eat and drink. Just because you can consume it doesn't mean you should. I might not be a health guru, but through life's lessons, I've learned a thing or two. Learn from my experiences for your own health's sake.

Fast forward to January 2023, the start of my weight loss journey leading up to my 25th wedding anniversary. My wife's back from the Philippines for a six-week stint before heading there again to prep for our celebration. I've set myself a challenge: transform my body to fit into that suit in three months. It's a grind—I'll be clocking in extra hours to stack up that cash while shuttling my daughters to work and squeezing in workout time. Right now, it's all about watching what I eat. Let's see if I can make this happen—I'm all in!

So, if all goes well (fingers crossed), this book is hitting the shelves in 2023. It's been a five-year journey packed with research trials, and now, finally, all that wisdom's going into print.

Achieving anything worthwhile takes effort, right? That's the truth. No shortcuts—just putting in the work.

I'm not some expert selling magic fixes or pricey programs you see on TV. Give it a try if you want; maybe it's your thing. If not, at least you'll learn something along the way.

It's all about finding strength within and staying positive. This book is your guide to a healthier you.

Think of life as a series of experiments. We make mistakes, we learn, and that's how we grow. But sometimes, we forget that failure is a crucial part of progress. If we really want to improve, it's time to learn from our mistakes and keep moving forward. Every day is a chance to get better.

Often, we're the ones holding ourselves back—whether it's in health, success, or relationships. The obstacles? Mostly in our minds. Blaming others might be easy, but deep down, it's all on us. When you look in the mirror at the end of the day, it's your choices, your wins, and your losses staring back at you.

Our lives are shaped by the decisions we make. "Sink or swim," "now or never"—these phrases are reminders. Remember Nike's "Just Do It"? It's classic. We all stumble, but what matters is getting up after each fall. Failure is normal; don't let it stop you. I always remind myself, "Maybe it's a sign," or if today doesn't go well, "Tomorrow's a new chance." So, hit that reset button and let's take on the challenge again.

To stay focused:

- Determination
- Discipline

- Focus
- Know your why?
- Committed

Listening to motivational speakers, favorite tunes, or inspiring movies—it all helps. Sometimes, even recalling the past serves as my motivation. Anything uplifting can make the journey smoother; just remember, the climb can feel steeper before it gets better.

Flipping through the earlier entries in this journal got me thinking. My exercise routines have changed over time and adapted to my schedule's whims. And guess what? It got tougher. My situation demands more motivation now. Imagine getting just 4 hours of sleep five days a week. And in that sliver of time, I've got to squeeze in my workout to stay fit and lose weight. Juggling responsibilities— dropping off one daughter at work, grabbing a few hours' sleep, picking her up, and then shuttling my other daughter. It's a hectic cycle that I've got to keep up for five weeks, hoping for a bit more sleep once things settle.

Starting slow is the plan. Build back stamina and regain strength—it's a step-by-step journey. Staying positive, staying motivated, and offering prayers are essentials here. Gratitude's key, too; health's the real treasure amidst life's shifts.

This book aims to guide those struggling with weight loss and old habits that need kicking.

Think about it: soda might not seem bothersome now, but it can bring trouble down the line. Research it yourself; soda's linked to diabetes and obesity. Tennis legend Andre Agassi once showed his fridge full of Coca-Cola in an interview. He's a favorite of mine, and I feel if he took better care of himself, he'd have a longer career. Similar story with basketball star Allen Iverson, who retired young due to health neglect. But there's someone like LeBron James—my favorite—still playing in the NBA at 38. Reports suggest he invests millions annually in self-care, diet, and using tech for muscle recovery. He's a shining example of investing in one's health.

On February 6, I embarked on my weight loss journey, clocking in at 180.03 pounds with a goal to shed 20 pounds in 3 months. The strategy: a mix of dieting, exercising, and intermittent fasting. Dieting means cutting back on food and sugar intake, while exercising includes running, walking, abs workouts, and lifting weights. But my schedule makes it a Herculean task—I'm averaging only 4 hours of sleep five days a week, chauffeuring both daughters to work and back, plus managing household chores. It's challenging, but where there's a will, there's a way.

I've mentioned it before, but I'm relying on protein powder, creatine, and BCAA 2:1:1 to fuel me for workouts and aid muscle recovery. It's not obligatory, but it does wonders for muscle repair and energy, especially given my diet.

One week down, no weigh-in today (February 12, 2023). My focus? Working out. These truncated sleep hours—five days a week—are no joke. Even on my days off, there's overtime to cover errands to run—it's a whirlwind. March 12 can't come soon enough. Both daughters switching to 2nd shift means I'll finally catch up on sleep and exercise properly.

Fast forward to February 18, almost two weeks into this regimen. It's a struggle with my jam-packed schedule, but looking at the numbers, it's promising. Shedding almost two and a half pounds weekly puts me on track to surpass my monthly goal of 10 pounds. Fingers crossed, but the key is to remain focused, stay motivated, and above all, avoid any injuries.

Now, on February 27, the hard work's paying off visibly. My weight's not drastically different, but I sense my fat turning into muscle. I feel stronger, and my midsection's definitely slimming down—a major win. The muscle soreness from the initial weeks is subsiding. By this 3rd week, my muscles are adapting to the consistent workouts.

Even more impressive: I'm handling 200 pounds during deadlifts and shrugs, which feels like progress. Hopefully, this trajectory will keep up. And here's a bonus—I'm not craving junk food or sugary drinks. It's a crucial part of this weight loss journey—remember the analogy with the drug addict's withdrawal period? That's the intensity of cutting out the bad stuff.

Exercise more + eat less = weight loss.

Yesterday, on March 4, 2023, I hit a roadblock. I felt weak and couldn't muster the energy to work out, so I chose to let my muscles rest the entire day. The day before, I was pushing heavy weights, and maybe that took a toll. But today, I feel rejuvenated, back on my feet, and lifting weights again. The lesson? Expect those bumps along the way, take a break, and then hit the gym with fresh determination.

Today marks March 7, 2023. After four weeks of committed weight loss efforts, I stepped on the scale: 171 pounds. A drop of 9 pounds averages at 2.5 pounds per week. I could've shed more if I'd managed better sleep. Just 4.5 hours a night isn't sufficient for muscle recovery. Still, I pushed through, sneaking in exercise whenever possible, sometimes just half an hour, sometimes a full hour.

In five days, I'll finally return to a regular sleep schedule, aiming for at least six hours a night. Optimism fuels me—I'm eyeing a 10-pound loss this March, a push toward my goal. Staying focused and motivated is key. Down 9 pounds, I feel good, but I'm not content yet. Those stubborn belly fat and love handles need to go.

Once again, this book is for those seeking a healthier lifestyle and weight loss. Let this be your guidepost, your blueprint to return to if you lose your way. Remember, as the MANDALORIAN said, "This is the way."

And today, on March 8, 2023, I hopped on my treadmill, and it felt fantastic. I upped my speed a bit, feeling lighter. It's a reminder—even when feeling weak days ago, never stop the workout grind. It's just a hump to get over. Keep at it. Stay dedicated, motivated, and determined to be better. Focus on your goals.

Losing weight and staying healthy—it's a marathon, not a sprint. Those habits we've held onto for ages don't vanish overnight. It's a gradual shift. If, say, you're used to smoking or drinking daily, start by cutting back to six days, then down to five, and so forth. Treat this change like a life-saving mission—because it is.

For me, it boils down to our daily habits: what we eat, drink, and do regularly. Binge-watching TV or gaming won't lead us to optimal health. Dedicate some effort, just as you would with anything else. Nothing's impossible. Consider it an investment in your health. A small commitment of half an hour to an hour daily keeps the doctor away.

Today, March 20, 2023, my old foot injury resurfaced four days ago, and boy, is it painful. I can walk, but running is out. Then, to add to the fun, a nasty allergy hit, courtesy of spring. The bottom line is no workouts for four days. Prior to falling ill, I was cutting back on food, and I think that's why I feel so drained. I'm planning to eat again to regain strength and resume workouts. My feet and allergies are about 90% better today, so it's workout time tonight. Unsure about the running part, but I'll give it a shot. My next day off isn't for three weeks, so pacing is key. Despite not overeating these past days, I've gained 5 pounds—mostly water weight. It's astounding how quickly the weight creeps up, but I'm not giving up. I believe I've got this.

Fast-forward to March 22, 2023. Yesterday marked my return to exercise. Battling pollen allergies and a bothersome right foot, I suspect my weakened state was due to not eating enough. My body couldn't keep up with the physical demands. Burning through calories, protein, and fats left me drained. Perhaps the allergy played a part, too. But adding more food, the healthy kind, revitalized me. Energy's back, and I've got to remember: exercise needs fuel. When I say more food, I mean nutritious choices, not junk. This book serves as my reminder—of the rights and wrongs on this journey.

Exercise is like waiting for a delayed package while eating feels like an instant delivery.

Exercise embodies delayed gratification while eating offers instant satisfaction.

As of March 31, 2023, I finally got back into the exercise groove after a hiatus. But, oh boy, my allergies kicked in, and while my weight's holding steady, my love handles and abs aren't showing much love. With just over a month left to hit my goals, I'm crossing my fingers, hoping no more sick days are ahead.

At work, I've had chats with colleagues in my age bracket battling health issues—from weight problems to troublesome gallbladders. If only they had my book to guide them on a healthier path.

Turning dreams into reality always takes a bit of sweat and grit.

Fast forward to April 11, 2023—let's talk progress. The pound down since March 31, 2023. Why only a pound? Well, the journey to weight loss is no sprint; it's a marathon. It took ten weeks for my body and mood to settle into this 10-pound loss. Feeling great, no grumpiness, no signs of being under the weather. Now, I'm eyeing another seven pounds off in three weeks. Keep the faith and keep pushing!

Why don't I weigh myself every day, you ask? My mantra is "Exercise matters more than the scale." Remember, exercising is a slow-cooked meal, not a fast-food fix. Weight loss doesn't happen overnight. Ten weeks to adapt to 10 pounds lost—that's the game. Imagine the shift for a 20-pound victory! Shifting bad habits for the right path is a journey, not a race. It takes time but promises a healthier, happier you in the end.

Remember, our most valuable treasure is our health. Money can't undo the toll of time. Invest in your health now, gather wisdom, and upgrade yourself. Don't wait until your retirement to wish you'd started earlier. Start living healthy today, so when retirement knocks, you're celebrating life, not popping pills for past neglect of your well-being.

The last time I updated this was on April 11, 2023. Fast forward to today, June 20, 2023. So, about that challenge, I set for myself back in April to shed 20 pounds... I got halfway there and then hit a roadblock when I went on a month-long vacation. No excuses; it was tough. I kept falling ill, and my job demanded a lot, not to mention juggling the kids and home. But I didn't stop trying, and that's the key.

Now that I'm back from vacation, work's ramped up to five, sometimes six days a week, clocking in 10-hour shifts. I need some serious motivation to get back on that treadmill. I know the drill for getting fit and healthy, so I'm just going to dive right in, starting slow and building myself up.

Being mindful of your health is crucial. Your mind steers your actions. When that tempting treat or drink pops up, no one's stopping you from indulging, but moderation is key. Yeah, I know, it's frustrating!

I haven't checked the scale in two weeks since my vacation, but I've got a hunch I might've gained 5 to 8 pounds. Tonight, after work, it's straight to the gym for me to kickstart things.

Here's a fun find: while shopping at one of my favorite stores, I stumbled upon this resistance band. Figured I could use it during downtime at work. Got this X-shaped resistance band, and it's been a game-changer. It lets me mimic my home workout routine at the office. Spending an hour or two with this every day is making a visible difference.

Do you know what drives me? Seeing some of my co-workers, younger than me, dealing with weight issues and already reliant on meds. That's the exact path I'm determined not to tread when I hit 62 and retire.

I have come to the conclusion that continuing this journal is gonna be redundant, so we have stab lists the foundation to be healthy, but just to summarize what I have learned during this journey:

- Change your "OLD BAD HABITS"
- We have to have a mindset of our self-goal. Focus.

- What food not to eat and what to eat.
- What drink not to drink and what to drink.
- When to eat and when to stop to eat.
- Diet, exercise, and intermittent diet.
- Know the correct form when exercising and know the wrong form when exercising.
- Never stop learning.
- Know your "WHY"

SELF-DISCIPLINE

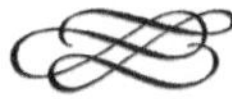

Self-discipline embodies the power to steer one's emotions and conquer vulnerabilities, to persist in what's right despite temptations to stray. The dedication to maintaining a healthy diet showcased remarkable resolve and self-discipline.

Here's a habit I highly recommend tailored to your situation: when you return home from work, engage in something you truly enjoy. In my own experience, coming back at night, I'd prefer hitting the treadmill and catching a show on TV until I drift off. Sometimes, I'd find myself mindlessly snacking while watching TV until I dozed off. This falls under the umbrella of habits we shape to foster better health.

This is my tested-and-true weight loss formula, honed over six years. It's been my go-to, and there's no reason it shouldn't work. Rushing weight loss might just lead to gaining it back and then some.

I advocate for everyone to maintain a journal chronicling their weight loss journey. It's been personally helpful, and I believe it can be a boon for others, too.

OTHER FACTORS

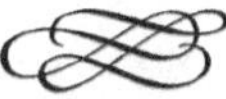

Remember, mere diet and exercise won't solely secure your health; a positive outlook is paramount. Be steadfast in your faith, irrespective of your beliefs. Embrace love, discard negativity, hate, and fear. These emotions can corrode your health, fostering illness. Pursue what you love, as happiness often correlates with a longer life. Don't be preoccupied with others' opinions; focus on steering your own mind. Authenticity matters—accept yourself while striving for improvement, whether through online resources or libraries.

For me, being healthy doesn't just mean a fit body but also a healthy mind. Mental well-being holds as much significance as physical health—where your mind goes, your body follows.

Remember, the choice between waking up happy or sad is in your hands. Your brain dictates which path you'll tread. As for me? I choose happiness.

There are various factors that could negatively impact your health: your environment, genetic predisposition, geographic location, work setting, family dynamics, relationships, and unforeseen circumstances—areas you might want to explore further.

Your environment, whether urban or rural, can influence your health. If you feel your surroundings are detrimental to your well-being, consider options for a change.

Genetic predisposition is pretty straightforward: personal hygiene matters. Skipping showers might keep you looking good but smelling otherwise, which isn't advisable.

Your geographical location might not always directly impact your health, but extreme weather conditions, for instance, could affect your physical and mental well-being.

Work environments can significantly affect health. If a job causes heightened stress anxiety or negatively impacts your health, it might be time to seek alternatives that prioritize your well-being.

Family dynamics can sway between healthy and challenging. Open communication about concerns is crucial—after all, family is meant for support.

Relationships, though wonderful, could turn toxic. If they adversely affect your mental health or daily life, it might be time to reassess and consider moving on.

Unexpected factors, like allergens in your living space or certain foods, could impact health. Be vigilant and address any unforeseen elements that could compromise your well-being.

Regarding exercise, it's best to research and tailor workouts to suit your body's needs—whether for your abs, legs, or arms. There's a plethora of options to explore and learn from.

Maintain an open mind and be receptive to new ideas. Experience often teaches by trying and learning from different approaches.

CONCLUSION

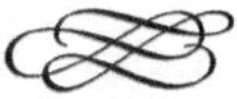

Lastly, as we age, our metabolism changes. Moderating food intake becomes crucial, so it's wise not to overeat and adjust eating habits as needed.

Sharing what I've learned feels like passing on a torch, lighting the way for others to navigate their own health journey.

You hold the power to make a world of difference.

Regular blood work and a chat with your doctor—these simple steps can unlock vital insights into your health. Never dismiss what your body might be trying to tell you; your doctor's guidance can be a game-changer.

This book feels like a living document, constantly growing. But there's a limit, and it's meant to guide, not dictate. Your health path? That's your canvas to paint. No one-size-fits-all; it's about finding what suits you best. So explore, learn, and prioritize your well-being.

Stay hungry—for knowledge, for a better you.

This journal is for those wrestling with a healthier lifestyle. Here's to a life teeming with joy and wellness. Many thanks, and stay tuned for more from me in "Suicide" and "Life." Your support means the world.